The Autoimmune Plant Based Cookbook

For Beginners

Author

Lidia J. Early

Contents page

INTRODUCTION

According to medical historians, autoimmune disease was first recognized in the mid-twentieth century by the scientific and medical communities. However, autoimmune disorders such as sympathetic ophthalmia and endophthalmitis phacoanaphylactica had been proposed much earlier. Affective disease was considered biologically implausible in the first half of the twentieth century. To emphasize that autoimmunity would go against nature's aversion to self-injury, Paul Ehrlich coined the term horror autotoxicus. The first indications that the immune system could self-harm were the discoveries of allergy and anaphylaxis. The immune system's ability to distinguish foreign from self, a process eventually understood in the context of immune tolerance, was a major roadblock in understanding the pathogenesis of autoimmunity. Researchers studying sympathetic ophthalmia and phacoanaphylactic endophthalmitis were in a good position to disprove horror autotoxicus, but they lacked sufficient experimental and clinical evidence to do so. In the 1950s, groundbreaking studies of chronic thyroiditis and a slew of clinical laboratory breakthroughs helped autoimmune disease gain widespread acceptance. The difficulties that ophthalmic researchers face provide insight into the development of medical concepts. We look at how ocular immunology contributed to the conceptualization of autoimmune disease and why it took so long to catch on.

Autoimmune diseases are a group of at least 80 illnesses that all have the same pathogenesis: an immune-mediated attack on the body's own organs. A total of 20 million Americans, primarily women, are affected by autoimmune disease. In industrialized countries, many diseases are becoming more prevalent. The treatment of autoimmune disease improved dramatically in the second half of the twentieth century, but progress has been hampered by the fact that the disease frequently progresses before a clinical diagnosis can be made. Prospective prediction using systems biology tools is the focus of research in the twenty-first century.

What Is An Autoimmune Disease, and How Do I Know If I Have One?

A condition in which your immune system attacks your body by mistake is known as autoimmune disease. Normally, the immune system protects you from bacteria and viruses. When it detects the intruders, it dispatches an army of fighter cells to attack them.

The immune system can normally distinguish between foreign and native cells. The immune system misidentifies parts of your body, such as your joints or skin, as foreign in autoimmune diseases. Autoantibodies are proteins that attack healthy cells and are released by the body. Only one organ is targeted by some autoimmune diseases. The pancreas suffers from type 1 diabetes. Diseases that affect the entire body, such as systemic lupus erythematosus (SLE), are examples.

The immune system attacks the body for a variety of reasons.

The cause of the immune system malfunction is unknown to doctors. However, some people are at a higher risk of developing an autoimmune disease. According to one study, women are more likely than men to develop autoimmune diseases, with 6.4 percent of women and 2.7 percent of men developing autoimmune diseases. The disease frequently begins during a woman's reproductive years (ages 15 to 44).

Certain ethnic groups have a higher prevalence of autoimmune diseases. African-Americans and Hispanics, for example, are more likely than Caucasians to develop lupus. Multiple sclerosis and lupus are examples of autoimmune diseases that run in families. Although not every family member will develop the same disease, they will all be predisposed to autoimmune disease.

Because autoimmune diseases are becoming more common, scientists believe that environmental factors such as infections and exposure to chemicals or solvents may play a role.

Another possible cause of autoimmune disease is a "Western diet." Inflammation is thought to be linked to the consumption of high-fat, high-sugar, and highly processed foods, which may trigger an immune response. This, however, has yet to be established. The hygiene hypothesis was the subject of a 2017 study. Children today aren't exposed to nearly as many germs as they were in the past thanks to vaccines and antiseptics. Their immune system may be prone to overreacting to harmless substances as a result of their lack of exposure.

The exact cause of autoimmune diseases is unknown to scientists. It's possible that genetics, diet, infections, and chemical exposure are all factors.

Autoimmune Diseases That Affect a Large Number of People

A total of 80 autoimmune diseases have been identified. Listed below are 14 of the most common.

Diabetic type 1

Insulin, a hormone produced by the pancreas, aids in blood sugar regulation. The pancreas' insulin-producing cells are attacked and destroyed by the immune system in type 1 diabetes mellitus.

Blood vessels, as well as organs such as the heart, kidneys, eyes, and nerves, can be damaged as a result of high blood sugar levels.

Rheumatoid arthritis (RA) is a type of inflammatory arthritis that affects the joints (RA)

The immune system attacks joints in rheumatoid arthritis (RA). The joints become red, hot, sore, and stiff as a result of this attack.

Unlike osteoarthritis, which typically affects people as they get older, RA can strike in your 30s or even earlier.

3. Psoriasis/psoriatic arthritis

Skin cells normally grow and then shed when they're no longer needed. Psoriasis causes skin cells to multiply too quickly. The extra cells build up and form inflamed red patches, commonly with silver-white scales of plaque on the skin.

Up to 30 percent of people with psoriasis also develop swelling, stiffness, and pain in their joints. This form of the disease is called psoriatic arthritis.

4. Multiple sclerosis

Multiple sclerosis (MS) damages the myelin sheath, the protective coating that surrounds nerve cells, in your central nervous system. Damage to the myelin sheath slows the transmission speed of messages between your brain and spinal cord to and from the rest of your body.

This damage can lead to symptoms like numbness, weakness, balance issues, and trouble walking. The disease comes in several forms that progress at different rates. According to a 2018 study, about 50 percent of people with MS need help walking within 15 years after the disease starts.

5. Systemic lupus erythematosus (SLE) (SLE)

Although doctors in the 1800s first described lupus as a skin disease because of the rash it commonly produces, the systemic form, which is most the common, actually affects many organs, including the joints, kidneys, brain, and heart.

Joint pain, fatigue, and rashes are among the most common symptoms.

6. Inflammatory bowel disease

Inflammatory bowel disease (IBD) is a term used to describe conditions that cause inflammation in the lining of the intestinal wall. Each type of IBD affects a different part of the GI tract.

Crohn's disease can inflame any part of the GI tract, from the mouth to the anus. Ulcerative colitis affects only the lining of the large intestine (colon) and rectum.

7. Addison's disease

Addison's disease affects the adrenal glands, which produce the hormones cortisol and aldosterone as well as androgen hormones. Having too little of cortisol can affect the way the body uses and stores carbohydrates and sugar (glucose) (glucose). Deficiency of aldosterone will lead to sodium loss and excess potassium in the bloodstream.

Symptoms include weakness, fatigue, weight loss, and low blood sugar.

8. Graves' disease

Graves' disease attacks the thyroid gland in the neck, causing it to produce too much of its hormones. Thyroid hormones control the body's energy usage, known as metabolism.

Having too much of these hormones revs up your body's activities, causing symptoms like nervousness, a fast heartbeat, heat intolerance, and weight loss. One potential symptom of this disease is bulging eyes, called exophthalmos. It can occur as a part of what is called Graves' ophthalmopathy, which occurs in around 30 percent of those who have Graves' disease, according to a study.

9. Sjögren's syndrome

This condition attacks the glands that provide lubrication to the eyes and mouth. The hallmark symptoms of Sjögren's syndrome are dry eyes and dry mouth, but it may also affect the joints or skin.

10. Hashimoto's thyroiditis

In Hashimoto's thyroiditis, thyroid hormone production slows to a deficiency. Symptoms include weight gain, sensitivity to cold, fatigue, hair loss, and swelling of the thyroid (goiter).

11. Myasthenia gravis

Myasthenia gravis affects nerve impulses that help the brain control the muscles. When the communication from nerves to muscles is impaired, signals can't direct the muscles to contract.

The most common symptom is muscle weakness that gets worse with activity and improves with rest. Often muscles that control eye movements, eyelid opening, swallowing, and facial movements are involved.

12. Autoimmune vasculitis

Autoimmune vasculitis happens when the immune system attacks blood vessels. The inflammation that results narrows the arteries and veins, allowing less blood to flow through them.

13. Pernicious anemia

This condition causes deficiency of a protein, made by stomach lining cells, known as intrinsic factor that is needed in order for the small intestine to absorb vitamin B-12 from food. Without enough of this vitamin, one will develop an anemia, and the body's ability for proper DNA synthesis will be altered.

Pernicious anemia is more common in older adults. According to a study, it affects 0.1 percent of people in general, but nearly 2 percent of people over age 60.

14. Celiac disease

People with celiac disease can't eat foods containing gluten, a protein found in wheat, rye, and other grain products. When gluten is in the small intestine, the immune system attacks this part of the gastrointestinal tract and causes inflammation.

A study noted that celiac disease affects about 1 percent of people in the United States. A larger number of people have reported gluten sensitivity, which isn't an autoimmune disease, but can have similar symptoms like diarrhea and abdominal pain.

Autoimmune Disease Symptoms

The early symptoms of many autoimmune diseases are very similar, such as:

fatigue achy muscles swelling and redness low-grade fever trouble concentrating numbness and tingling in the hands and feet hair loss skin rashes

Individual diseases can also have their own unique symptoms. For example, type 1 diabetes causes extreme thirst, weight loss, and fatigue. IBD causes belly pain, bloating, and diarrhea.

With autoimmune diseases like psoriasis or RA, symptoms may come and go. A period of symptoms is called a flare-up. A period when the symptoms go away is called remission.

Symptoms like fatigue, muscle aches, swelling, and redness could be signs of an autoimmune disease. Symptoms might come and go over time.

When to see a doctor

See a doctor if you have symptoms of an autoimmune disease. You might need to visit a specialist, depending on the type of disease you have.

Rheumatologists treat joint diseases, like rheumatoid arthritis as well as other autoimmune diseases like Sjögren's syndrome and SLE. Gastroenterologists treat diseases of the GI tract, such as celiac and Crohn's disease.

Endocrinologists treat conditions of the glands, including Graves' disease, Hashimoto's thyroiditis, and Addison's disease.

Dermatologists treat skin conditions, such as psoriasis. The Healthline Care tool can provide options in your area if you need help finding a specialist.

Test That Diagnose Autoimmune Diseases

No single test can diagnose most autoimmune diseases. Your doctor will use a combination of tests and a review of your symptoms and physical examination to diagnose you.

The antinuclear antibody test (ANA) is often one of the first tests that doctors use when symptoms suggest an autoimmune disease. A positive test means you may have one of these diseases, but it won't confirm exactly which one you have or if you have one for sure. Other tests look for specific autoantibodies produced in certain autoimmune diseases. Your doctor might also do nonspecific tests to check for the inflammation these diseases produce in the body.

A positive ANA blood test may be indicative of an autoimmune disease. Your doctor can use your symptoms and other tests to confirm the diagnosis.

How are autoimmune diseases treated?

Treatments can't cure autoimmune diseases, but they can control the overactive immune response and bring down inflammation or at least reduce pain and inflammation. Drugs used to treat these conditions include:

nonsteroidal anti-inflammatory drugs (NSAIDs), such as ibuprofen (Motrin, Advil) and naproxen (Naprosyn)

immune-suppressing drugs

Treatments are also available to relieve symptoms like pain, swelling, fatigue, and skin rashes.

Eating a well-balanced diet and getting regular exercise may also help you feel better.

The main treatment for autoimmune diseases is with medications that bring down inflammation and calm the overactive immune response. Treatments can also help relieve symptoms.

More than 80 different autoimmune diseases exist. Often their symptoms overlap, making them hard to diagnose. Autoimmune diseases are more common in women, and they often run in families. Blood tests that look for autoantibodies can help doctors diagnose these conditions. Treatments include medications to calm the overactive immune response and bring down inflammation in the body.

How to Get Started with an Autoimmune Diet

The general idea of the autoimmune diet is that you are removing any potentially inflammatory foods, but the specifics are a bit more difficult. Some sources consider foods like fruit and sweet potatoes OK, while others do not. For reference, some sources that I find most helpful are:

What to Eat

It can seem overwhelming, but this way of eating is actually relatively simple if you follow a template. My typical day on the autoimmune diet was:

Breakfast: A scramble of meat and cooked vegetables, a cup of homemade bone broth, some fermented vegetables, and supplements.

Lunch: A huge salad with leftover protein (meat, offal, or fish) and a small piece of fruit, a cup of bone broth, fermented water kefir or kombucha and olives.

Dinner: A stir-fry with some type of protein (meat, offal, seafood) with a lot of vegetables and allowed spices, evening supplements, and at least 1 cup of healthy starch like cooked winter squash, pumpkin, etc.

Avoiding These Foods

Grains: Rice, rye, quinoa, corn, oats, wheat, barley, and any other food or drink derived from grains.

Legumes: Black beans, pinto beans, lima beans, peanuts, soy, cocoa, lentils, and any other bean or legume.

Nuts and seeds: Almonds, chia, cashews, pecans, pistachios, and any other seed oil or product.

Select spices: Allspice, anise, pepper, poppy seeds, celery seed, cumin, caraway, mustard, nutmeg, and fennel seed.

Dairy and eggs: Milk, eggs, yogurt, cheese, cream, butter, and anything else made of dairy.
Nightshades: Bell peppers, eggplants, tomatoes, potatoes, cherries, red spices, goji berries, and tomatillos.

Processed/industrial foods: Additives and preservatives all contribute to an unhealthy gut lining, so anything that is store-frozen or packaged needs to go.

Sugars: molasses, brown sugar, regular sugar, and any foods containing sugar.

Alcohol: Beer, liquor, wine, and anything else containing alcohol (with the exception of kombucha).

Other Autoimmune Meal Plan Supplements

Diet is hugely important for all aspects of health, and for me, it became even more important after being diagnosed with autoimmune disease. It is by no means the only factor though. Personally, I found that these other things were equally important to recovery for me:

Sleep. It's my arch-enemy. I enjoy staying up late and sleeping little in order to accomplish more. This isn't good for my body. My health markers improve when I get at least 8-8.5 hours of sleep per night (blood tests, fasting blood sugar, etc). Here are a few sleep-related suggestions.

Reduction of anxiety Stress can have just as much of an impact on gut health and hormone levels as diet, which is another difficult one for me. Even with a healthy diet, I began to notice symptoms returning while working on my book. Use these techniques to help you manage stress and relax.

Supplements. I was hesitant to include this section because it won't help you at all if your diet, stress, and sleep aren't under control. After I'd optimized other factors, I discovered that certain supplements helped a lot. WP-Thyroid thyroid medication (under my doctor's supervision), Betaine HCL with protein meals, 5-MTHF and Methyl-B12, Probiotics, Fermented Cod Liver Oil, Cortisol support, Omega-3s, Vitamin D (daily sunshine in the morning), Magnesium, L-glutamine, Gelatin, and Vitamin C are some of the supplements I take. Before taking any supplements, I strongly advise you to consult with a good functional medicine doctor to determine your individual needs.

Move with care. You don't have to exercise vigorously, and it'll probably be difficult at first, but gentle exercise a few times a week can help with joint stiffness, digestion, and overall mood. A gentle swim, a slow-paced walk, or even some yoga can help your body recover.

Gratitude. Healthy thoughts are necessary for good health. To retrain your brain, relieve stress, and find peace with your body, try keeping a gratitude journal. It's incredible!

Support for Autoimmune Diets

This is a challenging diet. Pregnancy is, as well. Work and self-denial are sometimes required for the best things in life. The elimination phase is only temporary, but it provides insight into your own body and what foods you need to eat for optimal health.

Allowing it to stress you out will only make things worse. Allowing this to keep you awake at night isn't a good idea. Concentrate on nourishing and loving your body, as well as providing it with the building blocks it requires to function at its best. Encourage a friend or family member to accompany you on your journey for moral support if at all possible.

Meal Plan for an Autoimmune Diet

Because the AIP is so restrictive, it doesn't mean you can't eat well. For you, we've created a simple seven-day meal plan based on the elimination phase.

the first day

Banana, strawberry, and blueberry fruit salad for breakfast Lunch: arugula salad with oven-baked salmon and lemon slices Cucumber slices as a snack

Ground beef burgers for dinner

The second day

Sweet potato hash and steak for breakfast Avocado and turkey breast for lunch Snack: Beef jerky stick with sea salt Dinner: Asparagus with chicken thighs

3.

Sautéed ham with spinach for breakfast Chicken breast and kale chips for lunch. A can of tuna is a tasty snack.

Dinner: Mushroom burger (without the bacon).

The fourth day

Breakfast: Pork loin with a mushroom and onion mix

AIP chicken salad for lunch

Pickles, as a snack

Dinner: grilled tilapia with roasted squash and broccoli

The fifth day

Chicken livers with spinach for breakfast

Sandwiches made with turkey

Snack: A stick of beef jerky made in the Italian style.

Brussel sprouts and roasted duck for dinner

The sixth day

AIP porridge (breakfast)

Chicken poppers made with sweet potatoes for lunch Fresh melon with honey for a snack Dinner: Zucchini pasta with shrimp

The seventh day

Smoothie with blueberries and coconut Lunch: Asparagus with grilled chicken tenders Dry fruit as a snack

Coconut shrimp with grits for dinner

Recipes for Autoimmune Meals

1. Apple Pie That's Good for Your Autoimmune System

6 portions

Ingredients

5 peeled, quartered, cored, and thinly sliced Granny Smith apples 1 tbsp ground cinnamon + 1/2 cup coconut palm sugar 1 cup Arrowroot Flour 1/4 teaspoon Sea Salt + 1/4 teaspoon 1 lemon, juiced Coconut Flour (half cup)

3/4 cup organic cold-pressed coconut oil cold water, 1/2 cup

Process

Preheat the oven to 350 degrees Fahrenheit (180 degrees Celsius). If you haven't already done so, measure out your coconut oil and water and chill them.

In a big mixing bowl, put the apple slices. Bring enough water to a boil in a large pot to cover all of the apple slices. When the water is hot, pour it over the apples in the bowl until they are barely covered. Place them in a colander to drain and set aside while you prepare the crust.

In a medium mixing bowl, whisk together the arrowroot, coconut flour, palm sugar, and sea salt to make the crust. Cut the cold coconut oil into pea-sized lumps with a pastry cutter, butterknives, or your fingers. Gently mix in the cold water. Don't overmix the dough because it will be crumbly.

In a 9-inch pie dish, pour the mixture. Spread evenly across the surface with your fingers.

up the sides and down the bottoms. With a fork, prick some holes in the crust's bottom. The dough will behave differently than regular pie dough, and the less you handle it, the more flaky it will become. Bake for 15 minutes, then remove from the oven to cool while you prepare the filling.

Place the apple slices on a clean kitchen towel and blot them dry with it. In a large mixing bowl, whisk together the coconut palm sugar, cinnamon, and salt, then gently fold in the dry apple slices. Fill the crust with the mixture and arrange the slices as needed. Cook for 30-35 minutes, until the crust is golden brown, after sprinkling the pie with lemon juice.

Allow 10 to 15 minutes for cooling before serving.

Pork Chops in a Pan (AIP-friendly)

10 minute prep time 20 minutes total time 2 ppl

Ingredients

1 1/2 pound pork chops, bone in, two chops, 3/4 pound each 1 tablespoon of Primal Palate Super Gyro Seasoning

2 tablespoons lard (or other cooking fat of your choice) Tin Star Cultured Ghee (two tablespoons)

Thyme, fresh, a few sprigs 2 garlic cloves, crushed a quarter teaspoon of sea salt to serve as a finishing touch

Process

Allow pork chops to come to room temperature 15-20 minutes before cooking.

Allow the chops to rest after sprinkling them with Super Gyro seasoning.

Preheat the oven to 425 degrees Fahrenheit (200 degrees Celsius).

2 tablespoons of cooking fat, heated over medium heat in a medium cast iron skillet When the oil begins to shimmer, tilt the pan to coat it evenly and then add the pork chops.

Cook for 3:30 minutes on one side, then flip and cook for 3 minutes on the other. Flip for 2 minutes more, and then for 2 minutes more. This ensures that the sear is even.

Preheat the oven to 350°F and place the skillet inside. For a total of 10 minutes of roasting, flip the pork chops every two minutes.

Take the skillet out of the oven and place it on a cooling rack. Drain the fat from the skillet after removing the pork chops to a plate. Over medium heat, melt 2 tablespoons of cultured ghee. Sauté for a minute with the crushed garlic and thyme.

Return the pork chops to the hot pan and drizzle with ghee, thyme, and garlic. Cook for another minute, spooning the ghee over the chops as needed, before removing to serve.

Allow a few minutes for the pork chops to rest before seasoning with a coarse sea salt.

Serve immediately with a side dish of your choice.

Smoothie Recipe for "Brain Power"

5 minutes to prepare 5 minute total time 2 people

Ingredients

coconut milk, 2 cups

MCT oil (1 TBSP) or coconut oil (2 TBSP) gelatin powder, 2 tblsp

12 teaspoon extract de vanilla egg yolks (at least 2) ice, 1 cup

1 TBSP cocoa powder, 12 cup strawberries, 1 tsp cinnamon, and other flavors of your choice Optional 1 banana

Instructions

Blend all of the ingredients until smooth in a blender or Vitamix.

Smoothie Recipe with Cucumber, Melon, and Mint

5 minutes to prepare 5 minute total time 3 cups of serving

Ingredients

Cucumber, small

cantaloupe, 1 cup (cut into chunks) watermelon (1 cup) (cut into chunks)

12 c. mint leaves, fresh

1 quart of liquid (or coconut water)

Instructions

Cucumber, watermelon, and cantaloupe should all be peeled and diced.

Blend all of the ingredients until smooth in a high-powered blender. Enjoy the drink chilled or over ice!

4. Recipe for Tangerine Gummies

10 minute prep time 5 minutes to prepare 2 hours of chilling

2 hours and 15 minutes total time

8 people

Ingredients

1 cup tangerine juice from a fresh tangerine 14 cup honey 5 tbsp gelatin

Molded silicone 3/4 teaspoon powdered camu camu

4 drops essential oil of organic tangerine

Instructions

In a small sauce pan, whisk together the tangerine juice and honey until smooth.

Allow about 4 minutes for the gelatin to "bloom" on top of the juice mixture. Turn the heat to medium low when the top appears wrinkled and the gelatin has dissolved into the liquid.

Gently whisk for about 3-5 minutes, or until the gelatin has completely dissolved. If you go too far with this, the mixture will become extremely foamy.

Remove the pan from the heat and, if using, quickly whisk in the essential oil. This contributes to the citrus flavor being more prominent.

Fill your molds halfway with the juice mixture and chill until firm. An 8x8 glass baking dish will suffice if you don't have a mold. When the gelatin has cooled completely, simply cut it into squares.

Refrigerate the gummies after they've been made in a sealed container.

Recipe for Chia Seed Pudding

5 minutes to prepare

4 hours and 5 minutes in total

4 people

Ingredients

coconut milk, 2 cups

chia seeds, 12 cup

12 teaspoon extract de vanilla

14 cup maple syrup (or other sweetener of choice)

optional 14 tsp cinnamon

Instructions

To make the blended/smooth version, combine all ingredients in a blender and process on high for 1-2 minutes, or until completely smooth.

Blend all ingredients in a blender until smooth, including any added flavors, fruits, or chocolate, for the whole chia seed version. In a separate bowl, combine the chia seeds and the remaining ingredients.

Place the mixture in a jar or glass container in the refrigerator to gel for at least 4 hours or overnight.

To help it gel evenly, give it a few shakes or whisks within the first hour. I prefer to make this in the evening so that I can have it ready for a quick breakfast the next morning. It's also great to make ahead of time in the morning for a tasty pre-made dessert later in the evening.

Roasted Chicken Thighs with a "Super Gyro" Flavor

5 minutes to prepare

1 hr. 10 min. total 2 PEOPLE

Ingredients

Avocado Oil (1 tblsp.)

Garlic, 12 cloves 4 skinless chicken thighs 1 tsp Pinch Himalayan Pink Salt, Primal Palate Super Gyro Seasoning

Process

Preheat oven to 350 degrees Fahrenheit (180 degrees Celsius).

Sauté the garlic cloves for 2- 3 minutes (until the skins begin to brown) in a medium pot with the avocado oil over medium heat.

Sear the chicken thighs on both sides in a large skillet over medium high heat, about 2-3 minutes per side (do the skin-side first to avoid sticking).

Season the chicken with salt and the Primal Palate Super Gyro blend, then place it on top of the garlic. Preheat oven to 350°F. Cover and bake for an hour. Serve with a vegetable of your choosing.

8. Vegetables and Roasted Chicken

10 minute prep time

1 hr. 15 min. total 4 portions

Ingredients

1 pound frozen and cubed sweet potato, or a starchy vegetable of your choice

7/8 teaspoon salt, divided 2 tablespoons extra virgin olive oil

2 3/4 teaspoon Primal Palate Garlic and Herb Seasoning, divided or substitute your favorite seasoning blend

1 pound broccoli, florets (or substitute another vegetable) 3 Whole 1/2 pound of chicken

Process

Preheat the oven to 425 degrees Fahrenheit (200 degrees Celsius).

Toss sweet potatoes with 1 tablespoon olive oil, 1/4 teaspoon salt, and 1/2 teaspoon seasoning blend (or season to taste!) in a large mixing bowl. Place in a roasting pan's bottom.

1/8 teaspoon salt and 1/4 teaspoon seasoning blend for the broccoli Combine with the sweet potatoes in a roasting pan.

If desired, rinse and pat dry the chicken. 1 tbsp olive oil, 1/2 tsp salt, and 2 tsp seasoning blend should be massaged into the skin.

Place the chicken in the middle of the roasting dish after securing the legs and wings with kitchen twine. Breasts up, breasts down, breasts up, breasts down, breasts down, breasts down I'm aware that everyone has an opinion on this, so I'll let you decide. I cooked mine breast-up, but it may cook differently if you do it breast-down. You might want to move the vegetables from beneath the chicken to the pan's edges.

Bake for 45 minutes after covering the roasting pan with foil. The spices will not burn as a result. Remove the foil after 45 minutes and bake the chicken until it reaches a temperature of 165°F. Insert a meat thermometer into the meatiest part of the inner thigh to check for doneness, but make sure it doesn't touch the bone. After removing the foil, it will likely take an additional 20-30 minutes to fully cook.

Breakfast Bowls with Mashed Cauliflower

10 minute prep time 20 minutes total time 2 PEOPLE

Ingredients

Cauliflower (whole)

1 1/2 cup mushrooms or one 6 oz package mushrooms arugula, 4 cup

Bacon in 6 pieces

1/4 cup coconut milk (add 1 tablespoon at a time; you may not use all of it) 3 tblsp Amino Acids (Coconut)

1 tbsp Great Lakes brand unflavored beef gelatin 1 tbsp Yeast (Nourishment)

2 tablespoons bacon grease (I recommend reserving the bacon grease), but you can also use ghee, coconut oil, or avocado oil

Extra Virgin Olive Oil (1 tbsp) 2 teaspoons salt (or to taste)

Process

CAULIFLOWER, MASHED

Remove the leafy part of the stem from the cauliflower head and roughly chop it. Because the cauliflower will be steamed and blended, you can leave the rest of the stem in.

Using your preferred method, steam the cauliflower. A stovetop method is what I suggest.

Into a blender or food processor, add steamed cauliflower. You can also do this by hand or with an immersion blender, but I find that using a blender and food processor yields the best results.

1 Tbsp coconut milk, nutritional yeast (for a cheesy flavor), gelatin (for a thicker texture), about 1-2 tsp sea salt Start with 1 tablespoon of coconut milk, but depending on how much moisture is retained in your coconut, you'll probably need more.

cauliflower.

Until smooth, blend. Add a tablespoon of coconut milk at a time until you reach the desired consistency. Make sure the cauliflower is salted to your preference by tasting it.

MUSHROOMS, TO BE EXACT

Over medium low heat, heat the oil in a sauté pan.

Half-cut the mushrooms and toss them into the pan with the rest of the ingredients. To allow the flavors to fully develop, cook on low heat for a long time.

Pour in the Coconut Aminos once the mushrooms are fully cooked to deglaze the pan and caramelize the mushrooms on the outside.

While the glaze is still warm, remove it from the heat and sprinkle it with coarse sea salt.

BACON RECIPE

Preheat the oven to 375 degrees Fahrenheit (190 degrees Celsius).

Place the bacon on a baking sheet with a rim and parchment paper. 12-15 minutes until crisp

Remove the bacon from the pan and place it on a paper towel to cool. Extra grease will be absorbed. Save the grease that remains on the baking sheet in an airtight jar in the refrigerator to use later.

Roughly chop the bacon once it has cooled and store it until needed.

ASSEMBLY

Drizzle olive or avocado oil over the top of the ingredients in two bowls. Using coarse sea salt, season the dish. These ingredients can be prepared ahead of time and reheated for a quick breakfast bowl, or they can be eaten straight from the fridge.

Super Gyro Sliders from Delicata Squash

5 minutes to prepare 45 minutes total time

8 people

Ingredients

Grass-fed, 85 percent lean ground beef, 2 lb 2 Delicata Squash (wholesale)

1 tablespoon of Primal Palate Super Gyro Seasoning Bacon in 5 pieces

Avocado (whole)

Cilantro 4 sprig

Lime, whole

Himalayan Pink Salt, 1/2 teaspoon

Process

Preheat the oven to 400 degrees Fahrenheit (200 degrees Celsius).

Place your bacon strips on a sheet pan and place it in the cold oven to pre-heat while it cooks. Cook for 10-15 minutes, or until bacon is crispy.

When done to your liking, remove from the oven. Turn the oven off but leave the door open.

Set aside a ramekin filled with some of the fat from the sheet pan. On the sheet pan, leave about 2 tbsp

Make 1/2-inch rings out of your delicate squash. Remove the seeds using a spoon.

Place your rings on the greased sheet pan and flip them over to get bacon fat on both sides. 1/4 teaspoon salt, set aside

Preheat the oven to 350 degrees Fahrenheit and place the squash in it. 15 minutes of baking The rings should then be turned over gently. 5 minutes longer in the oven, or until fork tender.

Meanwhile, toss the ground beef, seasoning, salt, and bacon fat together in a large mixing bowl. 6–8 sliders should be formed.

Take the squash out of the oven and place it on a serving platter. Remove the squash from the sheet pan with a spatula and place it on a plate to cool.

Place the burger sliders on a sheet pan and bake for 15 minutes at 400 degrees F. Put a slider over each ring once they're finished.

Peel and mash your avocado. Over each patty, spoon a little more sauce.

Add a pinch of salt and a squeeze of lime juice to the tops. Add a few cilantro leaves on top for a finishing touch. Finally, top your sliders with 1/2-inch bacon chunks.

Mug Cake with Bananas (#11)

2 minutes to prepare 3 minute total duration

Ingredients

1 peeled and whole banana

1 tablespoon organic coconut oil (solid, not melted) Coconut Milk, 2 tbsp

Pure Vanilla Extract (1/2 teaspoon) Coconut Flour, 2 tbsp

1 teaspoon ground cinnamon Baking Soda (1/4 tsp)

Process

Add the coconut oil, coconut milk, and vanilla to the banana and mash it up. Combine the coconut flour, cinnamon, and baking soda in a large mixing bowl and thoroughly combine.

Fill a ramekin or a coffee cup halfway with the mixture.

Microwave for 3 minutes on HIGH (100%) power.

Allow to cool before eating.

Turmeric Tea, which is anti-inflammatory

2 minutes to prepare 10 minutes total time 1 portion

Ingredients

1 quart of liquid

Turmeric Powder (quarter teaspoon) 1/4 teaspoon ground cinnamon 1/4 teaspoon ground ginger 1/2 teaspoon raw honey

1 tablespoon of lemon juice

Process

Bring the water to a simmer in a small saucepan.

Stir together the spices, honey, and lemon juice. Cover the saucepan with a lid once it has been removed from the heat.

Allow 10 minutes for the ingredients to steam and combine.

Once cooled, take a drink. As you drink the tea, the spices will settle, so use a spoon to redistribute them.

Peach Mint Sauce Pork Tenderloin

10 minute prep time 25-minute total time 4 people

Ingredients

5 lb. fat-trimmed pork loin

1 sprig Mint Leaves, chopped 1/2 teaspoon Lemon Juice 2 whole peaches, skinned and diced

a quarter teaspoon of ground cinnamon

Process

Preheat the oven to 400 degrees Fahrenheit (200 degrees Celsius). Heat the pan over medium-high heat. Salt and pepper the pork tenderloins on both sides. Sear the tenderloin on both sides until brown in a hot pan. Remove from the pan and place in a baking dish once it has been properly seared. Bake for 25 minutes, or until an internal temperature of 150 degrees is reached.

Peaches should be diced while the tenderloin is cooking. In a small food processor, blend together the peaches, mint, lemon juice, and cinnamon until smooth.

Allow for 5 minutes of resting time on a cutting board after the tenderloin has been cooked. Cut and serve with the sauce once the meat has rested.

14. Pasta Salad (with Less Pasta) in the Summer

25-minute prep time 25-minute total time 8 people

Ingredients

2 Peeled and spiralized 1/2 pound yellow squash 6 oz Black Olives 1/2 cup sliced green onion 1/2 whole cucumber quartered and sliced

1 tbsp. Extra Virgin Olive Oil 3 Tbsp Apple Cider Vinegar, (for the dressing) (for the dressing) 1/2 tsp Garlic Powder, (for the dressing) (for the dressing)

3/4 tsp Onion Powder, (for the dressing) (for the dressing)

1 1/2 tsp Oregano, dried, (for the dressing) (for the dressing) 1/8 tsp Thyme, (for the dressing) (for the dressing)

1/2 tsp Basil, dried, (for the dressing) (for the dressing) 3/4 tsp Parsley, (for the dressing) (for the dressing)

3/4 tsp Sea Salt, (for the dressing) (for the dressing)

Process

Place all veggies in a large bowl.

Place all dressing ingredients in a small glass jar. Shake in mix thoroughly. Pour dressing over veggies and toss to combine.

Serve cold.

15. Tempura Shrimp

Prep Time: 30 minutes Total Time: 40 minutes 2 PEOPLE

Ingredients

3/4 cup Arrowroot Flour

1/4 cup Cassava Flour, plus 2 tablespoons 2 tsp Baking Powder

1/8 tsp Ginger, ground

Himalayan Pink Salt, 1/2 teaspoon

1/8 tsp Fish Sauce, about 3 drops 1 cup Sparkling Water\s2 Tbsp Coconut Aminos

Coconut Oil, Organic, Tropical Traditions steam refined coconut oil. Aim for at least 2 inches of oil in pot

2 lb Shrimp, Raw, wild caught, tail on

Process

Whisk together the dry ingredients in a large mixing bowl; only adding the 1/4 of cassava to start.

Pour in the fish sauce, coconut aminos, and sparkling water while whisking to combine. If batter is too loose, add a tablespoon of cassava at a time until the batter is about as thick as pancake batter (it should coat the whisk) (it should coat the whisk).

Choose a pot with high walls and a small diameter to maximize oil depth for frying. Add enough coconut oil (or lard, or your choice of cooking fat) to have a minimum depth of 3" of oil. Heat to 320 degrees Fahrenheit, monitoring the temperature with a candy thermometer.

Clean and peel the shrimp, removing all shell and only leaving the tail on. De-vein the shrimp.

Prepare a wire rack over a cookie sheet to allow fried shrimp to drain.

Dip the shrimp in the batter to coat, one at a time. Slowly lower into the hot oil, holding the shrimp by the tail, and allowing the batter to being to fry before releasing the shrimp. This will prevent the shrimp from sticking to the pot.

Working with only 2-3 shrimp in the pot at a time, cook the shrimp for about 3 minutes, until

the batter is golden brown. Place on a wire rack to drain. Repeat until all shrimp are fried.

16. Paleo Orange Teriyaki Meatballs

Prep Time: 20 minutes 25-minute total time 4 people

Ingredients

2 lb Chicken Breasts, boneless skinless, Ground 1/2 cup Green Onion, chopped

2 Tbsp Orange Zest

2/3 cup Orange Juice, fresh 2 tsp Ginger Root, minced 1/4 cup Coconut Aminos

1 Tbsp Apple Cider Vinegar 1 clove Garlic, minced

1 Tbsp Honey, Raw

Process

In a bowl, mix ground chicken (you can use any kind; breast or a blend) orange zest, pinch salt and green onions. On a parchment lined cookie sheet, form 2 1/2 inch sized meatballs. Bake at 350 until internal temperature reaches 170 degrees. Mine took about 30 minutes.

In a saucepan, add coconut aminos grated ginger, garlic, honey, vinegar and fresh orange juice. Bring to a simmer and reduce until sauce coats the back of a spoon. It will simmer for about 10 minutes and then start to watch it closely. It will start to foam and bubble as it is reducing and almost ready. You want the sauce to be the consistency of maple syrup.

When meatballs are cooked, place in a bowl and drizzle with the sauce. Gently toss to coat

all the meatballs.

17. Blackberry Cobbler

Prep Time: 15 minutes Total Time: 35 minutes Serves: 6

Ingredients

12 oz Blackberries

2 Tbsp Coconut Oil, Organic, plus more for greasing 3 Tbsp Water

1/4 cup Arrowroot Flour 1/4 cup Coconut Flour 1/4 cup Honey, Raw

1/4 tsp Salt

3/4 tsp Baking Soda 1 1/4 tsp Lemon Juice

Process

Preheat oven to 300. Lightly grease an 8×8 baking dish with coconut oil. Spread blackberries evenly in bottom of pan.

Mix remaining ingredients on medium speed until combined. Spread over blackberries. Bake for 35-40 minutes, until entire top is golden brown.

18. Warm Shrimp Salad with Bok Choy

Prep Time: 5 minutes Total Time: 10 minutes Serves 4

Ingredients

1 head Bok Choy, large 1/3 lb Shrimp, Raw

1/4 tsp Fish Sauce

3 Tbsp Coconut Aminos 2 clove Garlic

1/4 cup Watercress

Process

Heat a large skillet over medium-high heat.

Rinse the bok choy, and remove the large white veins near the bottom of each leaf. Chop the leaves lengthwise, and set aside.

Place the shrimp in the skillet, and stir in the fish sauce and coconut aminos. Sauté for 4-5 minutes.

Add the minced garlic and watercress, and continue to sauté until the shrimp is completely opaque.

Add the bok choy, and sauté 1-2 minutes, until it begins to soften slightly. Remove the skillet from the heat, and serve immediately.

19. Beets and Sweets Hash

Prep Time: 10 minutes Total Time: 45 minutes Serves 4

Ingredients

1 whole Sweet Potato, peeled and cubed to 1/4" pieces 1 whole Beets, peeled and cubed to 1/4" pieces

2 Tbsp Olive Oil, Extra Virgin 3 pieces Bacon, chopped

2 whole Green Onion, chopped

Process

Preheat oven to 375F

Coat potato and beet cubes with olive oil, salt and pepper Roast for 35-40 minutes until fork tender

Dice bacon and cook until crispy, drain fat reserving 1T

Add beets and sweets to the pan and heat together with bacon and reserved bacon fat Garnish with chopped scallions and serve

20. Turkey Breakfast Sausage (AIP friendly)

Prep Time: 2 minutes Total Time: 10 minutes Serves 4

Ingredients

1 lb Ground Turkey

1 Tbsp Primal Palate Breakfast Blend 1/2 Tbsp Lard

Process

Mix the ground turkey and spice blend in a bowl thoroughly. Form into patties by dividing the mixture in half, then in half again, and all portions in half one last time (giving you 8 small patties).

Heat the lard, or you choice of cooking fat, over medium heat in a skillet. Fry the patties about 4-5 minutes on each side, until fully cooked (may take 10 minutes, or longer, depending on the thickness.)

Serve alongside your favorite breakfast dishes!

21. Starch-Free Coconut Cream Pie

Total Time: 30 minutes Prep Time: 15 minutes Serves 8

Ingredients

1/2 cup Coconut Flour, (for the crust) 1/4 tsp Salt, (for the crust)

1/4 tsp Baking Soda, (for the crust)

3/4 tsp Cinnamon, ground, (for the crust)

1/3 cup Coconut Oil, Organic, melted (for the crust) 1/2 tsp Pure Vanilla Extract, (for the crust)

1/3 cup Honey, Raw, (for the filling)

2 tsp Gelatin, Unflavored, Knox brand, (for the filling)

1 cup Coconut, shredded, toasted at 350 for 5-6 minutes (for the filling) 16 oz Coconut Milk, (for the filling)

1/2 cup Coconut Butter, Organic, (for the filling) 1 1/2 tsp Vanilla Extract, (for the filling)

1/4 tsp Sea Salt, (for the filling)

Process

[For the crust] Preheat oven to 350.

In small bowl, whisk together dry ingredients: coconut flour, salt, baking soda and cinnamon. Set aside.

In stand mixer, beat wet ingredients together on medium. Add dry ingredients, mixing until fully combined.

Scrape dough into 9" pie plate. Place a piece of parchment paper (large enough to cover entire pie plate) over the crust. Using small hand-held rolling pin (or use a small drinking glass turned on its side), roll crust flat to cover the bottom and sides of the pie plate. The dough will thicken as the gelatin sets, so this may take some extra rolling compared to an egg-based crust.

Bake for 10-12 minutes, until golden brown. While crust is baking, toast coconut and prepare pie filling.

[For the filling] Toast coconut on a baking sheet for 5-6 minutes, until golden brown (Do not skip this step. Without it, the pie will be colorless and semi-translucent. It also adds great toasty flavor!)

In medium saucepan over medium heat, Whisk all ingredients together, except for the gelatin and toasted coconut.

Scoop out 2 teaspoons of the milk mixture and place it into a small dish. Add the gelatin and let it absorb the milk to create a rubbery mixture.

Cover the milk mixture and bring to a simmer. Whisk in rubbery gelatin mixture and whisk vigorously until the gelatin is completely dissolved. Turn off heat.

Stir in the coconut, and pour the mixture into the prepared graham pie crust.

Refrigerate for 4 hours, until completely cool and hardened throughout.

22. Slow Cooker Ham

Prep Time: 5 minutes Total Time: 4 minutes Serves 8

Ingredients

4 - 6 lb Ham

1/4 cup Honey, Raw 1/2 cup Orange Juice 2 tsp Rosemary, dried

4 Tbsp Coconut Oil, Organic 1 tsp Orange Zest

1 Tbsp Apple Cider Vinegar

Process

Place ham in slow cooker.

Put the rest of the ingredients on the ham. Cook on low for 4-6 hours.

23. Maple Brown Sugar N'Oatmeal

Prep Time: 10 minutes

Total Time: 40 minutes Serves 4

Ingredients

1 head Cauliflower, broken into 1-inch florets 4 Tbsp Coconut Oil, Organic, divided

3 Tbsp Coconut Milk

2 Tbsp Coconut Palm Sugar

2 Tbsp Maple Syrup, Pure, plus more for drizzling (optional) 1/4 tsp Sea Salt, heaping

1/4 tsp Cinnamon, ground, plus more for sprinkling (optional) 1 pinch Cloves, ground

Process

Preheat the oven to 425 degrees F. Line a large baking sheet with foil.

In a large, microwave-safe bowl, heat 2 tablespoons of coconut oil in the microwave until it's melted. Add the cauliflower florets and drizzle over 2 tablespoons of melted coconut oil. Toss the cauliflower florets and toss with your hands or a large spoon until the cauliflower is completely coated with oil.

Lay the florets in a single, even layer on the baking sheet. Place the baking sheet in the oven and roast the cauliflower for 20-25 minutes or until tender and the edges are turning a deep brown.

Remove the baking sheet from the oven and add the roasted cauliflower, 2 tablespoons coconut oil, coconut milk, sugar, maple syrup, salt, cinnamon, and cloves to the bowl of a large food processor. Process on high for 3 minutes, or 2 lb Chicken Breasts, boneless skinless, Ground 1/2 cup Green Onion, chopped\s2 Tbsp Orange Zest

2/3 cup Orange Juice, fresh 2 tsp Ginger Root, minced 1/4 cup Coconut Aminos

1 Tbsp Apple Cider Vinegar 1 clove Garlic, minced\s1 Tbsp Honey, Raw

Process

In a bowl, mix ground chicken (you can use any kind; breast or a blend) orange zest, pinch salt and green onions. On a parchment lined cookie sheet, form 2 1/2 inch sized meatballs. Bake at 350 until internal temperature reaches 170 degrees. Mine took about 30 minutes.

In a saucepan, add coconut aminos grated ginger, garlic, honey, vinegar and fresh orange juice. Bring to a simmer and reduce until sauce coats the back of a spoon. It will simmer for about 10 minutes and then start to watch it closely. It will start to foam and bubble as it is reducing and almost ready. You want the sauce to be the consistency of maple syrup.

When meatballs are cooked, place in a bowl and drizzle with the sauce. Gently toss to coat

all the meatballs.

17. Blackberry Cobbler

Prep Time: 15 minutes Total Time: 35 minutes 6 servings

Ingredients

12 oz Blackberries

2 Tbsp Coconut Oil, Organic, plus more for greasing 3 Tbsp Water\s1/4 cup Arrowroot Flour 1/4 cup Coconut Flour 1/4 cup Honey, Raw

1/4 tsp Salt

3/4 tsp Baking Soda 1 1/4 tsp Lemon Juice

Process

Preheat oven to 300. Lightly grease an 8×8 baking dish with coconut oil. Spread blackberries evenly in bottom of pan.

Mix remaining ingredients on medium speed until combined. Spread over blackberries. Bake for 35-40 minutes, until entire top is golden brown.

18. Warm Shrimp Salad with Bok Choy

Time to Prepare: 5 minutes 10 minutes total Serves 4 people

Ingredients

1 head Bok Choy, large 1/3 lb Shrimp, Raw\s1/4 tsp Fish Sauce

3 tbsp Amino Acids de Coco 2 clove Garlic

1/4 cup Watercress

Process

Heat a large skillet over medium-high heat.

Rinse the bok choy, and remove the large white veins near the bottom of each leaf. Chop the leaves lengthwise, and set aside.

Place the shrimp in the skillet, and stir in the fish sauce and coconut aminos. Sauté for 4-5 minutes.

Add the minced garlic and watercress, and continue to sauté until the shrimp is completely opaque.

Add the bok choy, and sauté 1-2 minutes, until it begins to soften slightly. Remove the skillet from the heat, and serve immediately.

19. Beets and Sweets Hash

Time to prepare: 10 minutes 45 minutes total Serves 4 people

Ingredients

1 whole Sweet Potato, peeled and cubed to 1/4" pieces 1 whole Beets, peeled and cubed to 1/4" pieces

2 Tbsp Olive Oil, Extra Virgin 3 pieces Bacon, chopped

2 whole Green Onion, chopped

Process

Preheat oven to 375F

Coat potato and beet cubes with olive oil, salt and pepper Roast for 35-40 minutes until fork tender

Dice bacon and cook until crispy, drain fat reserving 1T

Add beets and sweets to the pan and heat together with bacon and reserved bacon fat Garnish with chopped scallions and serve

20. Turkey Breakfast Sausage (AIP friendly) (AIP friendly)

2 minute prep time 10 minutes total Serves 4 people

Ingredients

1 lb Ground Turkey

1 Tbsp Primal Palate Breakfast Blend 1/2 Tbsp Lard

Process

Mix the ground turkey and spice blend in a bowl thoroughly. Form into patties by dividing the mixture in half, then in half again, and all portions in half one last time (giving you 8 small patties) (giving you 8 small patties).

Heat the lard, or you choice of cooking fat, over medium heat in a skillet. Fry the patties about 4-5 minutes on each side, until fully cooked (may take 10 minutes, or longer, depending on the thickness) (may take 10 minutes, or longer, depending on the thickness.)

Serve alongside your favorite breakfast dishes!

21. Starch-Free Coconut Cream Pie

Total Time: 30 minutes Prep Time: 15 minutes Serves 8 people

Ingredients

1/2 cup Coconut Flour, (for the crust) (for the crust) 1/4 tsp Salt, (for the crust) (for the crust)

1/4 tsp Baking Soda, (for the crust) (for the crust)

3/4 tsp Cinnamon, ground, (for the crust) (for the crust)

1/3 cup Coconut Oil, Organic, melted (for the crust) (for the crust) 1/2 tsp Pure Vanilla Extract, (for the crust) (for the crust)

1/3 cup Honey, Raw, (for the filling) (for the filling)

2 tsp Gelatin, Unflavored, Knox brand, (for the filling) (for the filling)

1 cup Coconut, shredded, toasted at 350 for 5-6 minutes (for the filling) (for the filling) 16 oz Coconut Milk, (for the filling) (for the filling)

1/2 cup Coconut Butter, Organic, (for the filling) (for the filling) 1 1/2 tsp Vanilla Extract, (for the filling) (for the filling)

1/4 tsp Sea Salt, (for the filling) (for the filling)

Process

[For the crust] Preheat oven to 350.

In small bowl, whisk together dry ingredients: coconut flour, salt, baking soda and cinnamon. Set aside.

In stand mixer, beat wet ingredients together on medium. Add dry ingredients, mixing until fully combined.

Scrape dough into 9" pie plate. Place a piece of parchment paper (large enough to cover entire pie plate) over the crust. Using small hand-held rolling pin (or use a small drinking glass turned on its side), roll crust flat to cover the bottom and sides of the pie plate. The dough will thicken as the gelatin sets, so this may take some extra rolling compared to an egg-based crust.

Bake for 10-12 minutes, until golden brown. While crust is baking, toast coconut and prepare pie filling.

[For the filling] Toast coconut on a baking sheet for 5-6 minutes, until golden brown (Do not skip this step. Without it, the pie will be colorless and semi-translucent. It also adds great toasty flavor!)

In medium saucepan over medium heat, Whisk all ingredients together, except for the gelatin and toasted coconut.

Scoop out 2 teaspoons of the milk mixture and place it into a small dish. Add the gelatin and let it absorb the milk to create a rubbery mixture.

Cover the milk mixture and bring to a simmer. Whisk in rubbery gelatin mixture and whisk vigorously until the gelatin is completely dissolved. Turn off heat.

Stir in the coconut, and pour the mixture into the prepared graham pie crust.

Refrigerate for 4 hours, until completely cool and hardened throughout.

22. Slow Cooker Ham

Time to Prepare: 5 minutes Total Time: 4 minutes Serves 8 people

Ingredients

4 - 6 lb Ham

1/4 cup Honey, Raw 1/2 cup Orange Juice 2 tsp Rosemary, dried

4 Tbsp Coconut Oil, Organic 1 tsp Orange Zest\s1 Tbsp Apple Cider Vinegar

Process

Place ham in slow cooker.

Put the rest of the ingredients on the ham. Cook on low for 4-6 hours.

23. Maple Brown Sugar N'Oatmeal

Time to prepare: 10 minutes

Total Time: 40 minutes Serves 4 people

Ingredients

1 head Cauliflower, broken into 1-inch florets 4 Tbsp Coconut Oil, Organic, divided\s3 Tbsp Coconut Milk

2 Tbsp Coconut Palm Sugar

2 Tbsp Maple Syrup, Pure, plus more for drizzling (optional) (optional) 1/4 tsp Sea Salt, heaping\s1/4 tsp Cinnamon, ground, plus more for sprinkling (optional) (optional) 1 pinch Cloves, ground

Process

Preheat the oven to 425 degrees F. Line a large baking sheet with foil.

In a large, microwave-safe bowl, heat 2 tablespoons of coconut oil in the microwave until it's melted. Add the cauliflower florets and drizzle over 2 tablespoons of melted coconut oil. Toss the cauliflower florets and toss with your hands or a large spoon until the cauliflower is completely coated with oil.

Lay the florets in a single, even layer on the baking sheet. Place the baking sheet in the oven and roast the cauliflower for 20-25 minutes or until tender and the edges are turning a deep brown.

Remove the baking sheet from the oven and add the roasted cauliflower, 2 tablespoons coconut oil, coconut milk, sugar, maple syrup, salt, cinnamon, and cloves to the bowl of a large food processor. Process on high for 3 minutes, or until the mixture is thick, creamy, and blended.

Spoon into bowls, top with cinnamon and maple syrup and/or fresh fruit (optional) and enjoy!2 lb Chicken Breasts, boneless skinless, Ground 1/2 cup Green Onion, chopped\s2 Tbsp Orange Zest

2/3 cup Orange Juice, fresh 2 tsp Ginger Root, minced 1/4 cup Coconut Aminos

1 Tbsp Apple Cider Vinegar 1 clove Garlic, minced\s1 Tbsp Honey, Raw

Process

In a bowl, mix ground chicken (you can use any kind; breast or a blend) orange zest, pinch salt and green onions. On a parchment lined cookie sheet, form 2 1/2 inch sized meatballs. Bake at 350 until internal temperature reaches 170 degrees. Mine took about 30 minutes.

In a saucepan, add coconut aminos grated ginger, garlic, honey, vinegar and fresh orange juice. Bring to a simmer and reduce until sauce coats the back of a spoon. It will simmer for about 10 minutes and then start to watch it closely. It will start to foam and bubble as it is reducing and almost ready. You want the sauce to be the consistency of maple syrup.

When meatballs are cooked, place in a bowl and drizzle with the sauce. Gently toss to coat

all the meatballs.

17. Blackberry Cobbler

Prep Time: 15 minutes Total Time: 35 minutes 6 servings

Ingredients

12 oz Blackberries

2 Tbsp Coconut Oil, Organic, plus more for greasing 3 Tbsp Water\s1/4 cup Arrowroot Flour 1/4 cup Coconut Flour 1/4 cup Honey, Raw

1/4 tsp Salt

3/4 tsp Baking Soda 1 1/4 tsp Lemon Juice

Process

Preheat oven to 300. Lightly grease an 8×8 baking dish with coconut oil. Spread blackberries evenly in bottom of pan.

Mix remaining ingredients on medium speed until combined. Spread over blackberries. Bake for 35-40 minutes, until entire top is golden brown.

18. Warm Shrimp Salad with Bok Choy

Time to Prepare: 5 minutes 10 minutes total Serves 4 people

Ingredients

1 head Bok Choy, large 1/3 lb Shrimp, Raw\s1/4 tsp Fish Sauce

3 tbsp Amino Acids de Coco 2 clove Garlic

1/4 cup Watercress

Process

Heat a large skillet over medium-high heat.

Rinse the bok choy, and remove the large white veins near the bottom of each leaf. Chop the leaves lengthwise, and set aside.

Place the shrimp in the skillet, and stir in the fish sauce and coconut aminos. Sauté for 4-5 minutes.

Add the minced garlic and watercress, and continue to sauté until the shrimp is completely opaque.

Add the bok choy, and sauté 1-2 minutes, until it begins to soften slightly. Remove the skillet from the heat, and serve immediately.

19. Beets and Sweets Hash

Time to prepare: 10 minutes 45 minutes total Serves 4 people

Ingredients

1 whole Sweet Potato, peeled and cubed to 1/4" pieces 1 whole Beets, peeled and cubed to 1/4" pieces

2 Tbsp Olive Oil, Extra Virgin 3 pieces Bacon, chopped

2 whole Green Onion, chopped

Process

Preheat oven to 375F

Coat potato and beet cubes with olive oil, salt and pepper Roast for 35-40 minutes until fork tender

Dice bacon and cook until crispy, drain fat reserving 1T

Add beets and sweets to the pan and heat together with bacon and reserved bacon fat Garnish with chopped scallions and serve

20. Turkey Breakfast Sausage (AIP friendly) (AIP friendly)

2 minute prep time 10 minutes total Serves 4 people

Ingredients

1 lb Ground Turkey

1 Tbsp Primal Palate Breakfast Blend 1/2 Tbsp Lard

Process

Mix the ground turkey and spice blend in a bowl thoroughly. Form into patties by dividing the mixture in half, then in half again, and all portions in half one last time (giving you 8 small patties) (giving you 8 small patties).

Heat the lard, or you choice of cooking fat, over medium heat in a skillet. Fry the patties about 4-5 minutes on each side, until fully cooked (may take 10 minutes, or longer, depending on the thickness) (may take 10 minutes, or longer, depending on the thickness.)

Serve alongside your favorite breakfast dishes!

21. Starch-Free Coconut Cream Pie

Total Time: 30 minutes Prep Time: 15 minutes Serves 8 people

Ingredients

1/2 cup Coconut Flour, (for the crust) (for the crust) 1/4 tsp Salt, (for the crust) (for the crust) 1/4 tsp Baking Soda, (for the crust) (for the crust)

3/4 tsp Cinnamon, ground, (for the crust) (for the crust)

1/3 cup Coconut Oil, Organic, melted (for the crust) (for the crust) 1/2 tsp Pure Vanilla Extract, (for the crust) (for the crust)

1/3 cup Honey, Raw, (for the filling) (for the filling)

2 tsp Gelatin, Unflavored, Knox brand, (for the filling) (for the filling)

1 cup Coconut, shredded, toasted at 350 for 5-6 minutes (for the filling) (for the filling) 16 oz Coconut Milk, (for the filling) (for the filling)

1/2 cup Coconut Butter, Organic, (for the filling) (for the filling) 1 1/2 tsp Vanilla Extract, (for the filling) (for the filling)

1/4 tsp Sea Salt, (for the filling) (for the filling)

Process

[For the crust] Preheat oven to 350.

In small bowl, whisk together dry ingredients: coconut flour, salt, baking soda and cinnamon.

Set aside.

In stand mixer, beat wet ingredients together on medium. Add dry ingredients, mixing until fully combined.

Scrape dough into 9" pie plate. Place a piece of parchment paper (large enough to cover entire pie plate) over the crust. Using small hand-held rolling pin (or use a small drinking glass turned on its side), roll crust flat to cover the bottom and sides of the pie plate. The dough will thicken as the gelatin sets, so this may take some extra rolling compared to an egg-based crust.

Bake for 10-12 minutes, until golden brown. While crust is baking, toast coconut and prepare pie filling.

[For the filling] Toast coconut on a baking sheet for 5-6 minutes, until golden brown (Do not skip this step. Without it, the pie will be colorless and semi-translucent. It also adds great toasty flavor!)

In medium saucepan over medium heat, Whisk all ingredients together, except for the gelatin and toasted coconut.

Scoop out 2 teaspoons of the milk mixture and place it into a small dish. Add the gelatin and let it absorb the milk to create a rubbery mixture.

Cover the milk mixture and bring to a simmer. Whisk in rubbery gelatin mixture and whisk vigorously until the gelatin is completely dissolved. Turn off heat.

Stir in the coconut, and pour the mixture into the prepared graham pie crust.

Refrigerate for 4 hours, until completely cool and hardened throughout.

22. Slow Cooker Ham

Time to Prepare: 5 minutes Total Time: 4 minutes Serves 8 people

Ingredients

4 - 6 lb Ham

1/4 cup Honey, Raw 1/2 cup Orange Juice 2 tsp Rosemary, dried

4 Tbsp Coconut Oil, Organic 1 tsp Orange Zest\s1 Tbsp Apple Cider Vinegar

Process

Place ham in slow cooker.

Put the rest of the ingredients on the ham. Cook on low for 4-6 hours.

23. Maple Brown Sugar N'Oatmeal

Time to prepare: 10 minutes

Total Time: 40 minutes Serves 4 people

Ingredients

1 head Cauliflower, broken into 1-inch florets 4 Tbsp Coconut Oil, Organic, divided\s3 Tbsp Coconut Milk

2 Tbsp Coconut Palm Sugar

2 Tbsp Maple Syrup, Pure, plus more for drizzling (optional) (optional) 1/4 tsp Sea Salt, heaping\s1/4 tsp Cinnamon, ground, plus more for sprinkling (optional) (optional) 1 pinch Cloves, ground

Process

Preheat the oven to 425 degrees F. Line a large baking sheet with foil.

In a large, microwave-safe bowl, heat 2 tablespoons of coconut oil in the microwave until it's melted. Add the cauliflower florets and drizzle over 2 tablespoons of melted coconut oil. Toss the cauliflower florets and toss with your hands or a large spoon until the cauliflower is completely coated with oil.

Lay the florets in a single, even layer on the baking sheet. Place the baking sheet in the oven and roast the cauliflower for 20-25 minutes or until tender and the edges are turning a deep brown.

Remove the baking sheet from the oven and add the roasted cauliflower, 2 tablespoons coconut oil, coconut milk, sugar, maple syrup, salt, cinnamon, and cloves to the bowl of a large food processor. Process on high for 3 minutes, or until the mixture is thick, creamy, and blended.

Spoon into bowls, top with cinnamon and maple syrup and/or fresh fruit (optional) and enjoy!until the mixture is thick, creamy, and thoroughly combined

Serve in bowls with cinnamon and maple syrup on top, as well as fresh fruit (if desired).

Spinach Chips with Sea Salt & Lime

5 minutes to prepare 30 minutes total time 6 PEOPLE

Ingredients

1 lime, 1 1/2 teaspoons zest + 2 teaspoons juice, divided 1/2 teaspoon salt

8 cup spinach leaves, whole, packed Extra Virgin Olive Oil, 2 tbsp

Process

Preheat oven to 275 degrees Fahrenheit (190 degrees Celsius). Use nonstick baking sheets or lightly grease two baking sheets. Rub together the zest and the salt in a small bowl with your fingers.

Toss the spinach with the olive oil in a large mixing bowl until it is well coated. Then toss in the lime salt, making sure each leaf gets a fair amount of it. If needed, use your hands.

Place the spinach in an even layer between the two cookie sheets you've prepared (do not crowd the leaves). 1 teaspoon lime juice in each batch

Bake for 30-35 minutes, or until the leaves are withered and very thin (time will vary depending on how fresh your spinach is, so keep an eye on it).

Before serving, remove the chips from the oven and cool completely on the pan.

Green Spritzer for the Holidays, No. 25

5 minute total time

2 PEOPLE

Ingredients

1 medium-sized cucumber 1 medium-sized lemon

Bartlett Pears, 3 oz.

3 large leaves of Kale, whole

16 oz. Sparkling Water 1 oz. Ginger Root, three-inch piece

Process

Remove the pears' cores and a portion of the lemon's rind.

In the juicer, combine the cucumber, lemon, pears, kale, and ginger.

Using a fine mesh sieve, strain the liquid. Pour one cup of juice concentrate into a tall glass filled with ice.

Add about a cup of club soda to the top and drink up! To taste, add more club soda or juice.

Rice with Cauliflower

10 minute prep time

7–9 minutes in total 4 people

Ingredients

1 garlic clove, chopped

1 tablespoon organic coconut oil

Cauliflower (one head)

a half cup of chopped yellow onion

To taste, 1/2 teaspoon Himalayan Pink Salt (and black pepper, if not following AIP)

1 teaspoon Primal Palate Garlic and Herb Seasoning (substitute 1/2 teaspoon Himalayan pink salt)

Process

Cauliflower should be rinsed and dried under cool water.

Grate the cauliflower with a cheese grater until it's coarsely grated (approximately the size of rice grains). To achieve the desired texture, pulse the cauliflower in a food processor.

In a skillet over medium heat, warm the coconut oil.

3–4 minutes, or until the onion is relatively translucent, sauté the onion and garlic. Continue to cook for another 4–5 minutes with the cauliflower rice.

Serve after seasoning with salt and pepper.

Glazed Salmon is number 27 on the list.

10 minute prep time 20 minutes total time 4 people

Ingredients

4 oz. wild-caught salmon filet (4 ounce filets) 1 teaspoon pure maple syrup

2 tblsp Amino Acids (Coconut) Warm water, 2 tbsp

Process

Preheat the oven to 350 degrees Fahrenheit (180 degrees Fahrenheit).

In a sauce pan, combine everything except the salmon.

Cook, stirring frequently, over medium heat until a glaze forms (5-7 minutes) Brush salmon filets with glaze and place on a baking sheet lined with parchment paper.

Bake for 20 minutes, or until the fish flakes easily when tested with a fork, pausing every 5 minutes to re-glaze. Green onions and sesame seeds can be added as a garnish.

Carob Chip Bars are number 28 on the list.

10 minute prep time 40-minute total duration 6 PEOPLE

Ingredients

2 peeled and chopped plantains Pumpkin Puree (half cup)

2 tablespoons flour (tigernut) Baking Soda (1/2 tsp.)

3 tbsp. organic coconut butter 1 tbsp. organic coconut oil

2 tbsp. raw honey

2 CUP COLD COCONUT MILK (ONLY THE CREAM)

Process

Preheat the oven to 350 degrees Fahrenheit (180 degrees Fahrenheit).

In a food processor bowl, combine all ingredients and process for a few minutes, or until smooth. Place in a loaf pan that has been greased.

1/2 cup carob chips, manually stirred in

40-50 minutes in the oven (until inserted knife comes out clean) Whip coconut cream in the meantime (i used my food processor)

Cool the bars on the counter for a few hours before putting them in the fridge. Refrigerate after topping with whipped cream.

Bison Stew (ninety-ninety-ninety

20-Minute Preparation 6 hours total 4 people

Ingredients

Medallions de bison de 2 lb 1 tablespoon organic coconut oil 3 sprig Thyme 2 cup celery, chopped

fresh rosemary sprigs 3 sprigs

1 quart Beef Broth (reduced sodium) 1 head Cauliflower, chopped 1 yellow onion, chopped

1/2 teaspoon salt (or more, depending on personal preference) (and black pepper, if not following AIP)

Process

In a cast iron skillet, brown bison stew meat on all sides in coconut oil. Transfer seared bison meat into a large soup pot.

Place chopped onion and celery into the pot with the bison. Pour beef broth over meat.

Season liberally with salt and pepper.

Place herbs, and celery greens into the pot, and turn burner onto medium heat. Bring stew to a boil, stirring often.

Once stew comes to a boil, turn heat down to low, and cover with a lid.

Simmer stew for 6-8 hours, adding the chopped cauliflower for the last hour of cooking.

30. One Pot Steamed Garlic and Herb Scallops with Veggies

5 minutes to prepare 10 minutes total time 2 PEOPLE

Ingredients

1/3 cup Water or broth

1 Tbsp Olive Oil, Extra Virgin 1 tablespoon of lemon juice

1 pinch Sea Salt 1/4 tsp Basil, dried

1/4 tsp Onion Powder or onion salt 1/4 tsp Garlic, minced\s6 oz Scallops, 1 serving (4-5 medium to large) (4-5 medium to large)

1 cup Kale, spinach, greens or favorite vegetables - chopped 2 Tbsp Greek Salad Dressing

Process

Place water and dash salt in small pot. Place steamer on top. In a separate bowl, toss your scallops in a bit of your favorite dressing (maybe 1-2 tbsp) and then add in your seasoning. Boil your water then Place scallops and veggies on top of steamer. Cover and steam with boiled water for 7-8 minutes or until scallops are opaque.

Remove from pot and place everything on plate. Add more seasoning and dash of lemon juice.

Scallops serve one but you can add more and make it serve two or more! Check scallops and veggies around 7-8 minutes to see if they are done.

Scallops are done when they are opaque in center and easy to slice, not chewy. You really can't undercook them.

If you are using smaller scallops, they will probably cook faster, around 5-6 minutes steamed.

31. Roasted Rosemary Beets

10 minute prep time 5 minute total time 2 PEOPLE

Ingredients

2 Tbsp Olive Oil, Extra Virgin

2 Tbsp Rosemary, fresh, chopped 3 Beets, chopped\s1/2 tsp Salt, (and black pepper, if not following AIP) (and black pepper, if not following AIP)

Process

Preheat the oven to roast at 400°F.

In a baking dish, toss beets in olive oil, salt, pepper, and rosemary.

Roast beets for 35 minutes or until crispy on the outside and tender in the center.

32. Slow Cooker Squash & Ground Beef Curry

10 minute prep time 6 hours total 6 PEOPLE

Ingredients

2 lb Ground Beef

1 whole Acorn Squash, cut into 1/2 inch cubes 13 1/2 oz Coconut Milk, (one can) (one can)

15 oz Pumpkin Puree, (one can) (one can) 1 1/2 cup Water

1 1/2 Tbsp Ginger Root, peeled and diced 5 cloves Garlic

1 whole Lemon, quartered 1/2 Tbsp Garlic Powder 1/2 Tbsp Onion Powder

1/2 Tbsp Turmeric Powder 1 tsp Cilantro, dried\s1 tsp Basil, dried 1 tsp Dill, dried\s1 tsp Cinnamon, ground 1/2 tsp Ginger, ground 1/4 tsp Cloves, ground\s1/2 cup Cilantro, (optional) for topping

Process

Break up the ground beef into small pieces, as small as you can make them.

Add the ground beef and all other ingredients (except the fresh cilantro) to your slow cooker.

Squeeze the lemons into the slow cooker before adding them.

Cover and cook on low for 4-6 hours or on high for 2-3 hours. If you're nearby, break up the chunks of ground beef halfway through the cooking time. If you're not, do so at the end.

Serve with cauliflower rice (you'll need about 1 1/2 - 2 cauliflower heads' worth of rice) and topped with fresh cilantro (optional) (optional).

33. Breakfast Stack

4 portions

Ingredients

4 slices AIP-friendly bacon 1 pound ground turkey

1 medium zucchini, grated coarsely

1/4 teaspoon dried sage Couple of pinches of salt Coconut oil (if needed) (if needed)

4 large flat mushrooms, stalks removed

2 medium avocados, stone and skin removed Juice of one small lemon

Rocket or watercress leaves

Instructions

Fry bacon in a large, dry skillet over medium heat until crispy. Set bacon aside. Leave fat in pan.

In a bowl, blend the turkey, zucchini, sage and a pinch of salt. Form into 6 patties.

Refrigerate 2 for a snack later; cook 4 now.

If there's not enough bacon fat in the skillet, add a little coconut oil. Cook patties 5-6 minutes per side. Check they are fully cooked throughout and then remove from pan and set aside.

Add mushrooms to skillet along with a splash of water. Cook for a few minutes each side, until they turn golden. Turn off the heat.

Quickly mash the avocado flesh together with a pinch of salt and the lemon juice.

To assemble: place the upturned mushroom on a plate and arrange a small tangle of the watercress or rocket leaves on top. Place the turkey and zucchini patty on top of that and finish with a spoonful of guacamole and a slice of bacon. Eat while hot.

34. Healing Breakfast Porridge

20 minutes total time Yield: 1-2

Ingredients

2–3 tbsp lightly toasted sunflower seeds (or 1 Tbsp tahini) - if you can tolerate. For seed substitute, use an additional 2 tbsp of coconut flakes or coconut butter (grounded)

2 tbsp unsweetened shredded coconut

1 tbsp chia seed or flaxseed (omit for AIP or substitute with 1 tbsp collagen/ gelatin powder)
1/2 tsp cinnamon

1 tsp ginger, ground Pinch of turmeric, ground Pinch of sea salt

1/2 cup water or coconut milk, more if needed

1 cup chopped squash, cooked (ex: butternut squash or kabocha/ or acorn squash). If using Instant pot you will need additional coconut oil or ghee and water

Pure maple syrup or raw honey

Extra toppings: berries or cherries, pomegranate seeds, coconut cream or coconut yogurt to top.

Instructions

Stove Top Instructions

Combine all dry ingredients (sunflower seeds, coconut chia, and spices and grind in a coffee grinder or blender until you get a flour-like consistency. If you are short on time, use tahini instead of sunflower seeds and just mix all together.

.

In a small bowl, add the dry mixture with water or coconut milk, let it adsorb and form a gel. Feel free to save a little bit of the gel for topping!

Scoop cooked squash and gel mixture into a blender and blend until smooth.

Heat the porridge stove-top on medium heat just until it starts to bubble. Stirring occasionally.

Remove from heat, pour into your favorite bowl, and top with the dry mixture you set aside.

Optional Add in –> 1 tsp of ghee if desired, helps improve digestion and healthy fats help absorb the nutrients adding in more nourishment.

Top with fresh berries, extra milk, etc.

INSTANT POT OPTION

Peel and Chop your squash into large pieces. Place in the instant pot with 1 tbsp or less of coconut oil. Add in a pinch of cinnamon and nutmeg and sauté for 5 minutes, turning the squash.

Once the squash is coated, add 1/3 cup of water to Pressure Cooker cooking pot and lock on lid, close pressure valve.

Cook on Manual High Pressure for 5-6 minutes.

Allow a 10 minute Natural Pressure Release. Or use a quick release if short on time. Release the lid, drain the water then puree the squash with a hand blender.

Mix in your other ingredients (dry mix and tahini/sesame mix) and a splash of milk (non-dairy). Stir all together. Place the lid back on and keep it on warm mode until ready to serve.

35. COCONUT CRUSTED COD WITH MANGO SALSA

25-minute prep time Cook Time: 10 minutes Total Time: 35 minutes Yield: 4-6 servings

INGREDIENTS

Salsa Ingredients

1 large mango, peeled and diced 1 avocado, cubed 1/2 small red onion, diced 1 cucumber, diced

1 bunch cilantro, chopped 2 cloves garlic, minced 1/2 teaspoon sea salt

1 tablespoon olive oil 1 lime, juiced

Fish Ingredients

24 ounces cod fillets, cut into 2 inch thick strips 1 1/2 cups coconut flour

1 1/2 teaspoons ginger powder 1/4 teaspoon sea salt

2 cups coconut milk

1 cup finely shredded coconut 2 tablespoons coconut oil Mango salsa INSTRUCTIONS

First prepare the mango salsa and set aside. Wash, dry, and debone the cod fillets.

Combine the coconut flour, ginger powder and salt on a plate or shallow bowl. Place the coconut milk in another shallow bowl, as well as the shredded coconut. Dip the cod strips into the coconut milk, then the coconut flour mixture, back into the coconut milk, and finally into the shredded coconut, paying special attention to creating a thick breading.

Heat the coconut oil in a large skillet on medium-high heat. When it is hot, cook the cod strips for five minutes a side depending on thickness of the fish, or until the top and bottom are nice and browned and the fish is cooked throughout. Once the cod strips are in the pan, try not to fuss with them too much because there is no egg in the breading, they are a little delicate.

Serve with mango salsa.

Conclusion

The AIP diet is designed to reduce inflammation by systematically removing all foods known to or believed to agitate autoimmune systems and the gut. It's split into two phases: the elimination phase and the reintroduction phase. By eating a strict, additive and irritant-free diet for at least thirty days, you can analyze how foods make you feel from a "clean slate".

Ideally, after you complete the AIP diet you will have a unique guide on which foods make you feel what ways and why. This is a powerful asset you can use to shape your health for years to come. While the science is still not conclusive on the AIP diet, early studies are promising.

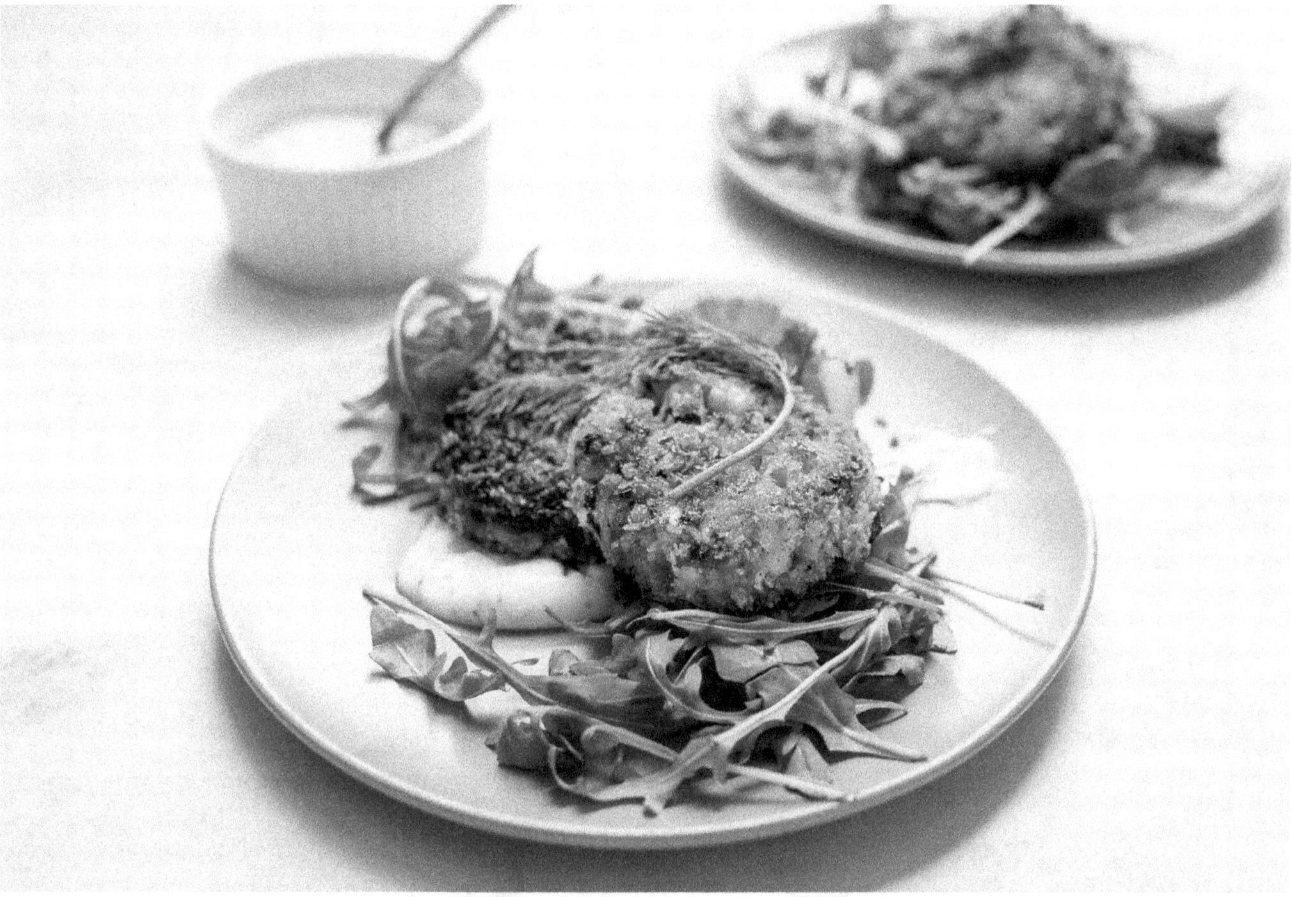

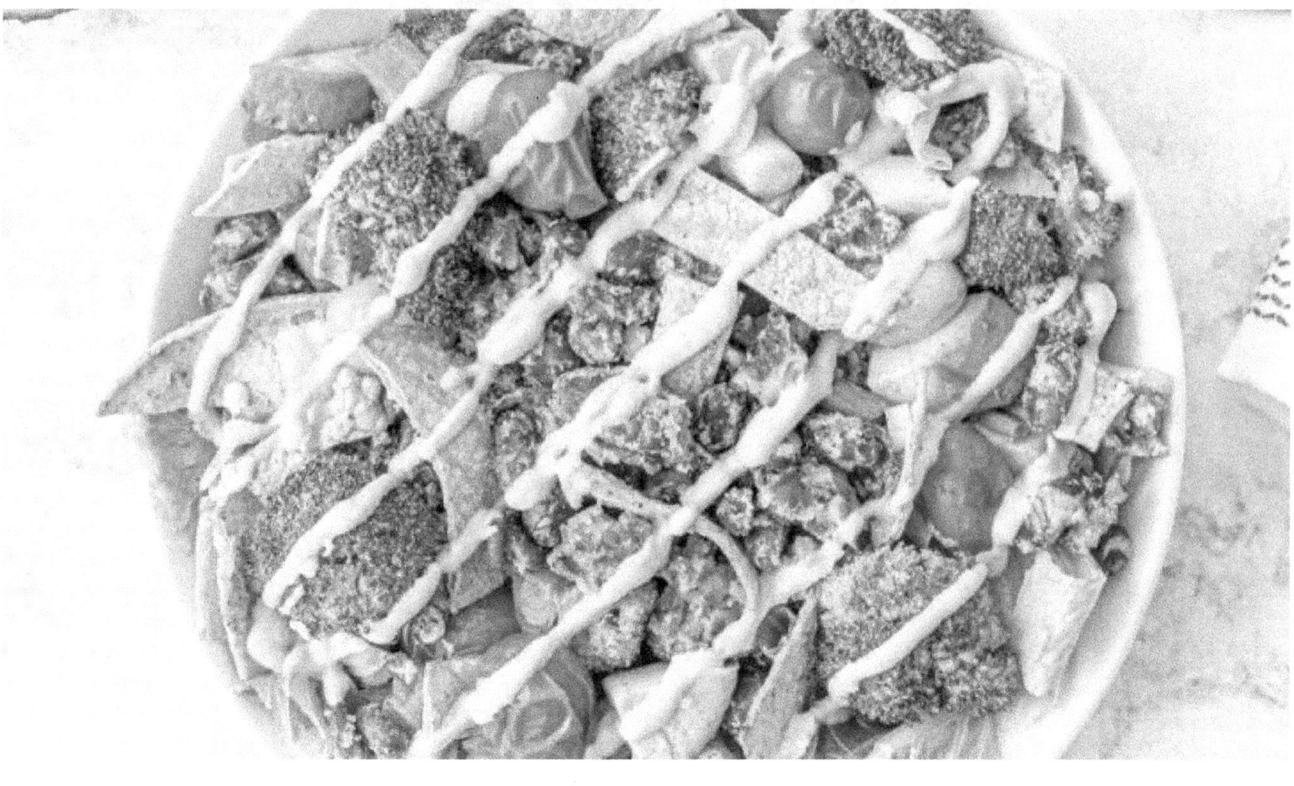

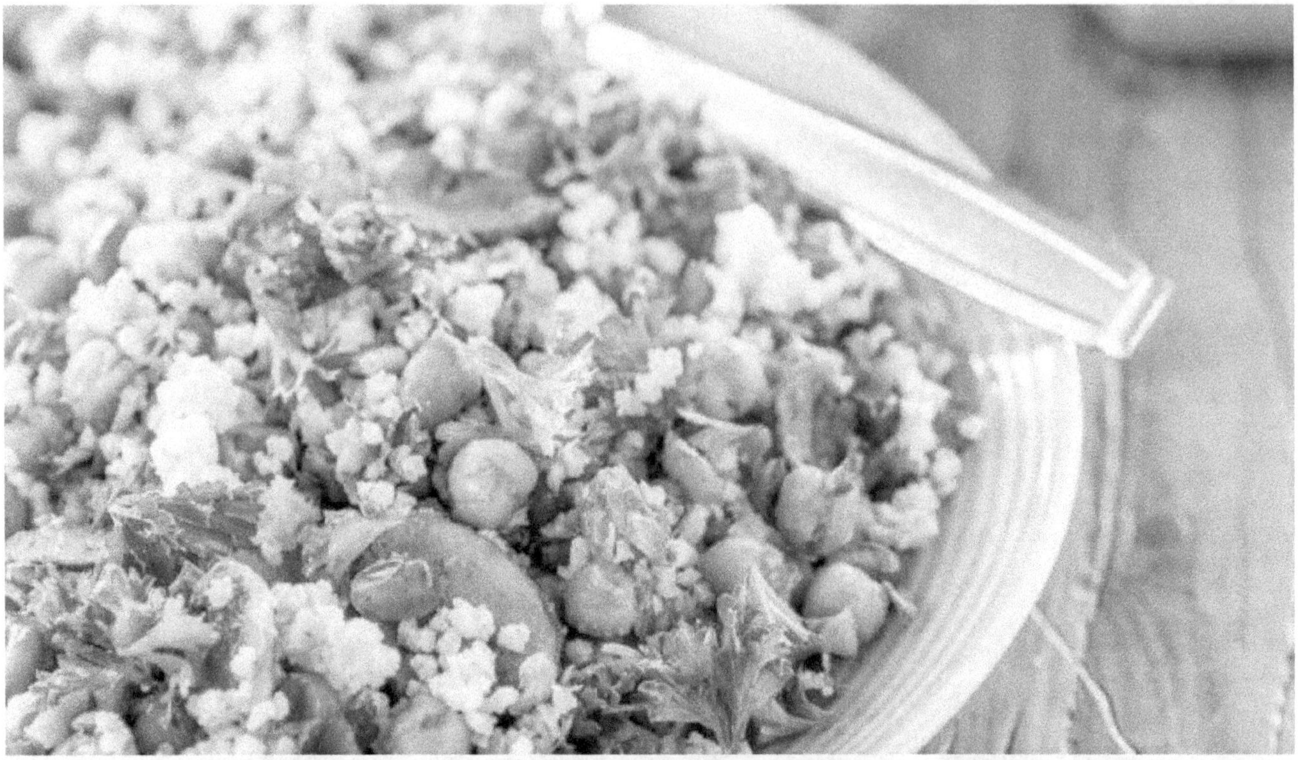

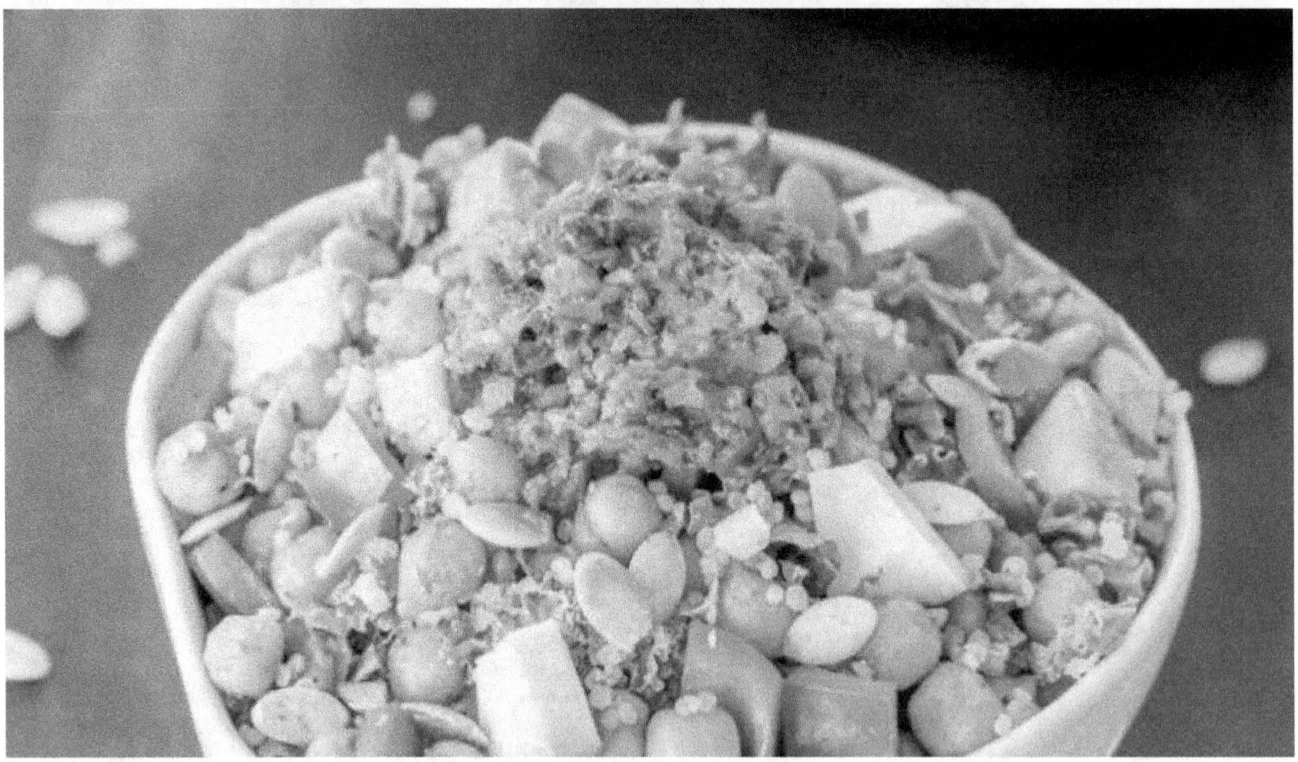

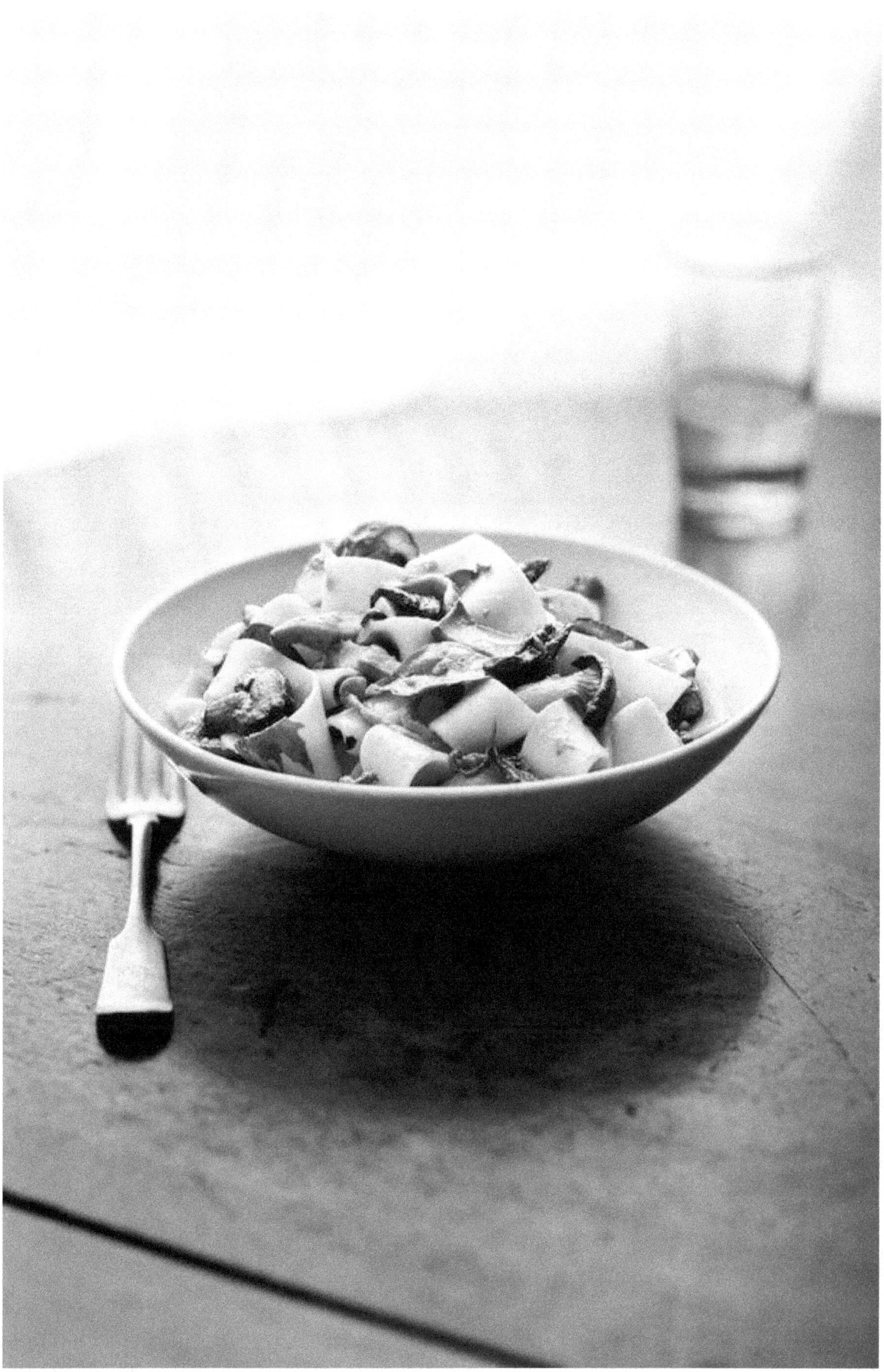

CPSIA information can be obtained
at www.ICGtesting.com
Printed in the USA
LVHW062113180122
708837LV00010B/485

9 781804 372029